The 2007 Pfizer Medical School Manual

A Practical Guide to Getting into
Medical School

Mike Magee, M.D.

The 2007 Pfizer Medical School Manual/Mike Magee, M.D.
104 p. 1 cm.
ISBN: 978-1-889793-21-4
Printed in Canada

The 2007 Pfizer Medical School Manual
is provided as part of the
Pfizer Medical Humanities Initiative,
a program which encourages
the development of humanistically
and scientifically balanced
physicians committed to
patients, families, and
their communities.

For more information about the
Pfizer Medical Humanities Initiative,
contact:
www.positiveprofiles.com
and
www.healthpolitics.org

Table of Contents

I
Introduction

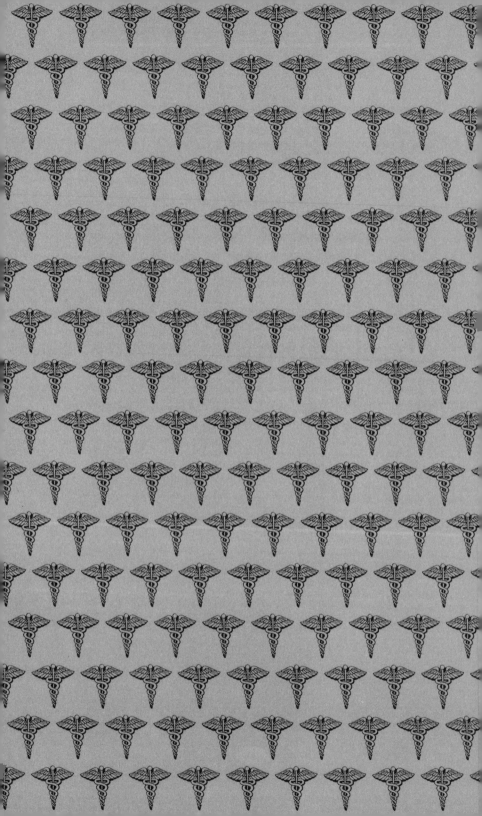

An Introductory Message by Author
Mike Magee, M.D.

*T*his book is dedicated
to those who seek to
devote their lives to
a career in medicine. It is
intended to assist would-be
physicians as they navigate
the complex and often
daunting medical school
admissions process.

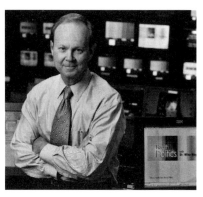

*In an era that heralds accelerated breakthroughs and scientific
discoveries, medical science is on the brink of an unprecedented
ability to understand and improve human life. Our understanding of the genetic and molecular mechanisms underlying diseases has greatly expanded the scope of the possible. Knowledge
of the genome will allow us to predict and prevent diseases
before they start. Future physicians can anticipate a constant
stream of newly minted medical advances to revolutionize their
medical practice, particularly the treatment of heart disease,
arthritis, diabetes, Alzheimer's and cancer.*

*Physicians who thoughtfully and passionately embrace this
medical and technological revolution will shape the future of
medicine. Medicine will also be shaped by demographic
changes. By 2030, 50% of American adults will be 50 or more
years old, and the population of adults over 85 years old will
have doubled. The challenge of meeting the ever-increasing
demand for quality health care will depend upon progress in*

scientific understanding and managing the complexity of four and five generation American families.

Through all the medical breakthroughs and demographic changes to come, our need for interpersonal connection will remain. Medicine will always be a profession that marries the role of medical mystery solver with compassionate healer. Medical schools will forever seek students who communicate effectively, who rigorously pursue intellectual excellence, and who find purpose, satisfaction and dignity in human service.

This book is not a secret formula that will guarantee admission to medical school. It does provide aspiring physicians with specific, practical recommendations that will help them positively and memorably present themselves to prospective medical schools.

In addition, I invite you to become part of my online community by subscribing to Health Politics (*www.healthpolitics.org*) and actively participating in my personal blog (*http://blog.health-politics.org/weblog/*). Both are available to you without charge.

With a call to those committed to transforming their knowledge of health and science into actions that will improve people's lives, and with wholehearted endorsement of your career choice, I urge tomorrow's physicians onward!

Sincerely,

Mike Magee ms

Mike Magee, M.D.
Host, Health Politics
www.healthpolitics.org

II

Overview

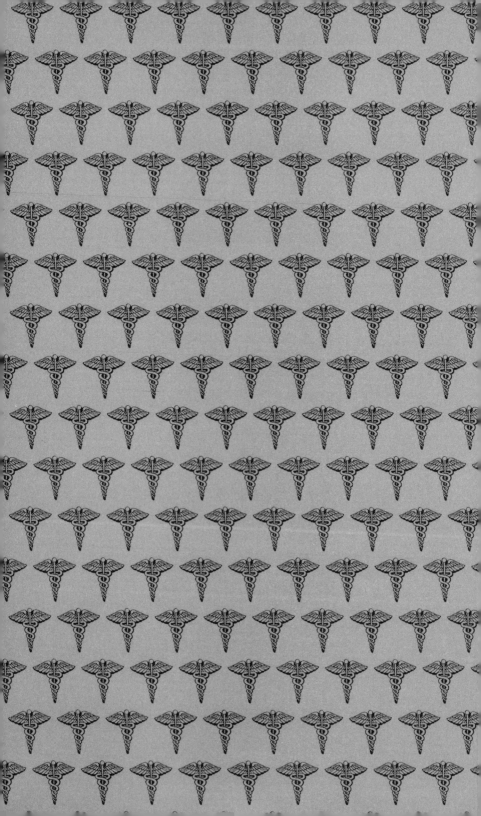

II Overview

There are approximately 81,749 students at any one time enrolled in America's 147 medical schools. Each year this unique body of talented and diverse individuals is revitalized with approximately 20,884 women and men chosen from more than 47,100 applicants. These medical students are highly qualified, having fulfilled exacting science requirements and achieved excellent grade point averages and MCAT scores.

With more than twice as many applicants as there are seats, how do medical schools decide whom to accept? Four criteria are used to evaluate applicants:
- Grade point average
- MCAT scores
- Letters of recommendation
- Interviews — often the determining factor in accepting or rejecting candidates.

As important as the interview is, preparation for it is often overlooked. The rigorous undergraduate science curriculum, the demanding process of choosing and applying to schools, the hours of study for MCAT exams, and the development of relationships with professors who will write insightful, personal letters of recommendation often take precedence over preparation for an admissions interview. Yet, successful interviews require research, introspection and analytical thought. Chapter IV of this manual prepares applicants for medical school interviews.

Undergraduate Preparation

Today, medical schools accept a broad range of undergraduate majors. Indeed, approximately 16% of applicants for the allopathic medical school Class of 2009 (who entered medical school in Fall, 2005) majored in the humanities and social sciences. The acceptance rate for liberal arts majors roughly mirrored the overall acceptance rate. Still, most applicants choose a traditional path, with approximately 71% of members of the allopathic medical school Class of 2009 majoring in the biological or physical sciences.

Most colleges and universities maintain a pre-medical advisory office. While advice on curricular choices varies from school to school, undergraduates should enroll in courses that will develop their competence in required sciences as well as contribute to their well-rounded candidacy.

Most medical schools require successful completion of the following laboratory courses:
- introductory biology (one year)
- inorganic or general chemistry (one year)
- organic chemistry (one year)
- physics (one year)

Other courses commonly required by medical schools include:
- calculus or college math or statistics
- English (one year)
- humanities electives

Some schools require or recommend one or more of

the following courses:
- anatomy and physiology
- biochemistry
- genetics
- psychology or behavioral science
- computer science

Since the MCAT test required for admission to medical school assesses your knowledge of science concepts and principles, as well as problem-solving, critical thinking and writing skills, complete these courses during the first three years of college so that by your junior year you can take the April or August MCATs.

Allopathic vs. Osteopathic Medical Schools

In the United States and its territories, 125 allopathic medical schools grant Doctorates of Medicine, or M.D.s, and there are currently 22 colleges of osteopathic medicine that offer the Doctor of Osteopathic Medicine (D.O.) degree (www.aacom.org/colleges/). Two of the colleges are provisionally accredited and are accepting applications for the class starting in August 2007. They are:
- A.T. Still University COM—Mesa, AZ
- Lincoln Memorial University—DeBusk COM, Harrogate, TN

The first school of medicine in the United States was founded at the University of Pennsylvania in 1765 by John Morgan, a young surgeon. In 1892, some 127 years later, Andrew Taylor Still, M.D., founded the first School of Osteopathic Medicine in Missouri. This school emphasized musculoskeletal training and manipulation to aid bodily function. Though chartered by state law to grant graduates an M.D., Taylor chose instead to grant Doctorates of Osteopathy, or D.O.s.

Over the next century, the two branches of medicine often clashed. By 1974, the federal and state government as well as the American Medical Association recognized both M.D.s and D.O.s as legally separate but equal branches of medicine. Today, allopathic and osteopathic medical schools share the following characteristics:

- Applicants possess four-year undergraduate degrees and meet similar science prerequisites
- Accepted students must complete four years of medical school, including two years of didactic and two years of clinical experience
- Graduates may pursue specialist or generalist tracks
- Graduates must pass board exams for licensure
- Graduates are qualified to commence residency training programs in fully accredited hospitals

To learn how students enrolled in allopathic schools compared to those enrolled in osteopathic schools, see Chapter V, pages 55-56. To learn more about allopathic medical schools, contact the Association of American Medical Colleges at www.aamc.org. For osteopathic medical schools, contact the American Association of Colleges of Osteopathic Medicine at www.aacom.org.

Application to Medical School

Of the 125 accredited allopathic medical schools in the United States, 117 participate in the AMCAS program. The AMCAS (www.aamc.org/amcas) electronic application is available on the Web in May of each year. AMCAS processes and forwards your application and MCAT scores to the individual schools to which you are applying, beginning around July 1st. Application through AMCAS allows you to complete the application process once and to simultaneously apply to any of the 117 participating medical schools. The eight allopathic medical schools that will not participate in AMCAS for the 2008 entering class are noted below:

- University of Missouri-Kansas City School of Medicine
- University of North Dakota School of Medicine and Health Sciences
- Texas A&M University System Health Science Center College of Medicine
- Texas Tech University Health Sciences Center School of Medicine
- University of Texas Southwestern Medical Center in Dallas Southwestern Medical School[1]
- University of Texas Medical Branch at Galveston[1]
- University of Texas Medical School at Houston[1]
- University of Texas Medical School at San Antonio

[1] The M.D./Ph.D. program at this school is participating in AMCAS for the 2008 entering class.

The AAMCAS application fee is based upon the number of schools to which applicants apply. The fee for applications for the 2007 entering classes is $160 for the first designated school and $30 for each additional school, regardless of the point at which you add school designations. Those unable to pay this fee may apply for a waiver through the AAMC Fee Assistance Program (FAP). Visit the FAP website (www.aamc. org/fap) for additional information. In addition to this fee, individual schools have supplemental application fees that range from $20 to $130. Upon receipt of your AMCAS application, each school usually sends secondary application materials as well as a bill for the school's individual application fee. Failure to remit this fee may result in no further action being taken on your application.

To obtain an AMCAS web application (the paper version is no longer produced) or additional information about AMCAS, contact:

AMCAS
American Medical College Application Service
Section for Application Services
2450 N Street, NW
Washington, DC 20037-1123
(202) 828-0600
www.aamc.org

All osteopathic medical schools participate in a comparable application service. The American Association of Colleges of Osteopathic Medicine Application Service, or AACOMAS, processes and forwards your application and MCAT scores to the individual schools to which you apply beginning around June 1st.

To obtain an AACOMAS application, available in April, contact your college advisory office, AACOMAS participating schools, or AACOMAS at:

AACOMAS
American Association of Colleges of Osteopathic
Medicine Application Service
5550 Friendship Blvd.
Suite 310
Chevy Chase, MD 20815-7231
(301) 968-4190
www.aacom.org

The MCAT

The MCAT is a standardized multiple choice and written examination administered 22 times each year, in January and from April through September. Most schools recommend that the test, which is required for admission to medical school, be taken 12-18 months prior to intended enrollment. A Spring MCAT is recommended so that results are ready in time for your AMCAS and/or AACOMAS applications. While you may repeat the test, it is unwise to take the MCAT "just for practice" because all scores are included on your score report. It is best to do well on your first take.

The MCAT assesses facility with problem-solving, critical thinking, writing skills and knowledge of science concepts and principles prerequisite to the study of medicine. The MCAT is four-hours and twenty-minutes long with three additional, optional, 10-minute breaks. Its four components are:

- Physical Sciences, 52 questions, 70 minutes, a test of physics, and inorganic chemistry, concepts and problem-solving skills that includes graphs, tables and charts.

- Verbal Reasoning, 40 questions, 60 minutes, a test of reading comprehension, reasoning skills and critical thought. Content is drawn from humanities, social sciences and natural sciences.

- Biological Sciences, 52 questions, 70 minutes, a test of general biology and organic chemistry, DNA and genetics concepts and problem-solving skills that includes graphs, tables and charts.

- Writing Sample, two essay questions, 60 minutes, a test of writing and analytical skills.

Five scores are reported, one for each section and a combined Total. Verbal Reasoning, Physical Sciences and Biological Sciences grades are scored on a scale from 1 (lowest) to 15 (highest). The Writing Sample is scored on a scale ranging from J (lowest) to T (highest). In the Total score, the three numerical scores are summed and the Writing Sample score is appended, e.g., 45T.

The MCAT is an entirely computer-based test, administered worldwide. Information and registration can be found at www.aamc.org/mcat. The MCAT Practice Test Online provides Web access to more than 1200 authentic MCAT items through full-length MCAT Practice Tests, extensive diagnostic feedback, and bulletin boards for MCAT discussions. For more information, please visit www.e-mcat.com. One Practice Test is available free on that site.

Payment of approximately $210 covers administration of the MCAT exam and reporting of your test scores to schools. The $210 MCAT fee may be reduced for those with extreme financial need. Fee Reduction Program materials can be found at www.aamc.org/fap.

In addition to test preparation texts such as Arco's, Flower's, Baron's, Monarch's and Barnes and Noble's, students may find the following resources useful in preparing for the MCAT:

1. Association of American Medical Colleges
   MCAT – Student Manual
   Membership and Publication Orders
   (202) 828-0416
   www.aamc.org
   AAMC provides a student manual of sample tests.

2. Kaplan Inc.
   888 7th Avenue
   New York, NY 10106
   (800) KAP-TEST
   www.kaplan.com
   An MCAT review course is available.

3. Princeton Review
   2315 Broadway
   New York, NY 10024
   (212) 925-6447
   www.review.com
   An MCAT review course is available.

Early Decision Program

Two third's of U.S. allopathic medical schools participate in an Early Decision Program (EDP) for highly qualified applicants with a strong preference for one school. Applicants who participate in this program agree to apply to only one school and are required to await that school's decision prior to initiating applications to other schools; each school is required to inform all EDP candidates of its EDP admission decision by October 1. An applicant agrees, in advance, to enroll in the EDP school, if that school accepts him or her. Applicants not accepted at a school through EDP may be deferred for consideration with regular candidates, or rejected, by that school.

An applicant who is not accepted by the school to which he or she applied through EDP can submit an application to other schools immediately after having been notified of the outcome of the EDP application or, at the latest, on October 1st, the final date for notification of EDP decisions. However, since all application materials have already been completed and verified, they can immediately be distributed electronically to other medical schools of interest. In this instance, applicants should take care to meet the application deadlines for receipt of supplementary application materials by these schools. Some schools have mid-October deadline dates, but most school deadlines are in November or December. In 2005, approximately 47% of EDP candidates received an acceptance through EDP, with another 17% receiving at least one acceptance after October 1st through the regular admission process. Similarly, approximately 47% of regular applicants received an acceptance to at least one medical school during the regular application process.

Some osteopathic medical schools also have an Early Decision Program. Visit www.aacomas. aacom.org for more information.

Recommended Number of Applications

For the past several years, persons applying to allopathic medical schools submitted an average of 11 applications. Students applying to osteopathic medical schools submitted applications to an average of 6.5 medical schools.

The data indicate little significant difference in acceptance rates for those applying to multiple schools. For example, in 2005, applicants made application to an average of 12 allopathic medical schools. In recent years, the acceptance rates for applicants to a total of 11, 19, and 26 schools ranged from 52 to 58%. More important than acceptance rates is choosing schools that match your specific qualifications and interests and that have historically accepted students from your college.

A number of factors may enhance your chances for admission. These include state residency, institutions where you apply early decision or have an existing personal connection, and membership in a special interest group.

Selecting a Medical School

To decide upon a medical school, read available literature both from and about different schools, visit campuses and their web sites, and discuss schools with your advisors and with current medical students. 10 factors to consider when comparing schools are:
1. Policies favoring state residents
2. Size of student body
3. Student: faculty ratio
4. Patient care opportunities
5. Geographic location
6. Student services
7. Sources of financial support
8. Cost
9. Unique volunteer/research/leadership activities
10. Positioning for residencies or future graduate studies

Differences in curriculum should also be noted. 10 curricular areas expanding in American medical schools are:

1. Nutrition
2. Geriatrics
3. Epidemiology
4. Environmental health
5. Preventive and community health care
6. Medical humanities
7. Medical ethics
8. Clinical decision making
9. Medical information systems
10. Socioeconomics of medicine

Chances for admission may be enhanced if the following characteristics apply to you:

1. State resident
2. Member of a under-served group
3. Willingness to practice in under-served or rural areas
4. Plans to become a primary care physician
5. Existing relationship with school
6. Residence in adjacent, contractually linked states
7. Early submission of application
8. Your college is one of the medical school's "feeder" schools
9. Credentials comparable to or exceeding the school's applicant pool

III
The Application Process

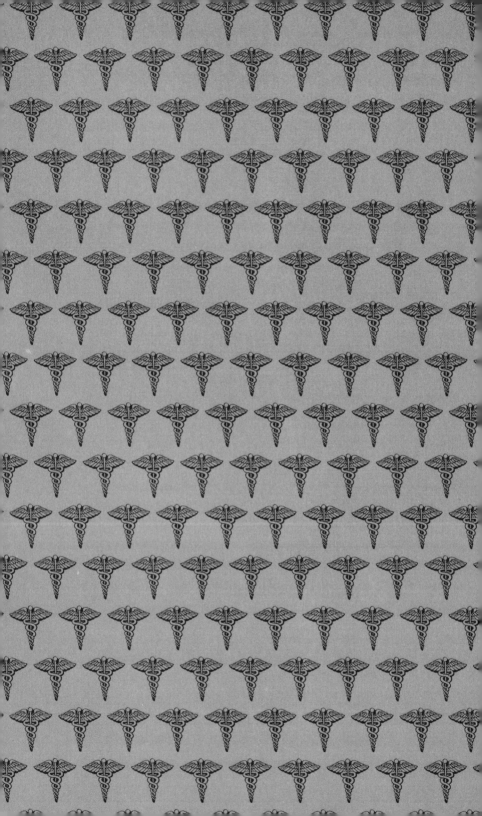

III   The Application Process

Calendar of Deadlines
Entering Medical School in 2008

MCAT
Beginning in January 2007, the MCAT will be administered only in a computerized format. There will be a total of 22 MCAT administrations in 2007. These administrations will occur on 19 different days during the months of January, April, May, June, July, August, and September. On three of these days, there will be two MCAT administrations, one in the morning and one in the afternoon. On the other 16 days, there will be either a morning or an afternoon administration. Registration for the MCAT and scheduling of a test administration will be completed online. Visit the MCAT Web site (www.aamc.org/mcat) for additional information about registration, scheduling, and score reporting.

Begin MCAT Review .... 3-4 months prior
to MCAT date

AMCAS Begins Accepting   On or about
Official Transcripts .... May 1, 2007

AACOMAS Begins Accepting
Official Transcripts .... May, 2007

AACOMAS Web Application Available ...... May, 2007

AMCAS Web Application Available .... May, 2007

AMCAS Submissions Begin .... June, 2007

AACOMAS Submissions Begin .... May, 2007

Early Decision Program   Prior to
Application Filed........................ August 1, 2007

Early Decision Application	
Complete	August 1, 2007
Early Decision Rendered	No later than October 1, 2007
Application Deadline for Most Medical Schools	Between October 15 and November 15, 2007

Timeline

Create a timeline by first deciding when you want to enter medical school. Then, in sequential order, follow these steps:

1. Fulfill science requirements

Basic undergraduate sciences in biology, chemistry and physics, including laboratories, are a prerequisite for application to medical school. To be competitive, you should attain A's and B's in these courses. By January of your junior year, request and verify the accuracy of transcripts from all colleges attended.

2. Volunteer or work in health settings

Most medical schools seek prospective students who have been exposed to physicians and patients in health-related settings. Such experience demonstrates your knowledge and commitment to health science and to human service. Interviews often aggressively explore just how significant your involvement was.

3. Broaden your course selection

If possible, take classes that will expand your potential as a caring individual, community leader and physician.

4. Develop onsite advisors

Cultivate strong relationships with faculty who can advise and support you. These relationships will surely enrich your academic experience.

Professors can recommend courses and appropriate medical schools and write letters of recommendation. Professors might also invite you to work with them on projects or in their labs. Meet with professors and advisors at least twice each semester to discuss your aspirations, intellectual passions and extracurricular activities.

5. Prepare for the MCAT

Generally, performance on the MCAT mirrors SAT performance. Home study programs or more formalized MCAT review courses can improve performance.

6. Take the Spring MCAT if possible

The MCAT exam is administered 22 times each year, January through September. A Spring MCAT allows scores to be delivered to AMCAS or AACOMAS in time for AMCAS and AACOMAS applications and affords the opportunity to repeat the test if necessary. The test should be taken 12-18 months prior to intended enrollment. For more information, contact MCAT at (319) 337-1357 or www.aamc.org.

7. Submit transcripts to AMCAS/AACOMAS

Transcripts require the greatest lead-time and should be requested, verified and sent prior to completion of your AMCAS, non-AMCAS or AACOMAS applications. Since official transcripts are accepted by AMCAS, AACOMAS and non-AMCAS schools when the application becomes live for that processing season, you should request that each school you have attended send you a transcript. Check each transcript for accuracy and then ask each school to send a single, official transcript to AMCAS or AACOMAS and an official transcript to each of your non-AMCAS participating schools.

Applications for AMCAS and AACOMAS are generally available in May and submissions begin around June 1. For information regarding application to allopathic medical schools, contact AMCAS at (202) 828-0600 or www.aamc.org. Application information regarding non-AMCAS schools must be obtained directly from these schools. For information regarding application to osteopathic medical schools, contact AACOMAS at (301) 968-4190 or www.aacom.org.

8. Submit applications early to optimize your chances

Early applications are associated with higher acceptance rates and greater likelihood of being invited for interviews. Submit applications as soon as possible and include your scores, transcripts, personal essay and letters of recommendation. Maintain records of all your applications.

9. Monitor application submission

Track the arrival of your applications to ensure their completeness and their receipt by each school to which you are applying. To assume safe delivery is to court disappointment. You must be your own best advocate in the application process.

The Admissions Committee and Its Function

In most medical schools, the Admissions Committee is comprised of 15 or more members of the general faculty, as well as representatives from the medical student body. The Dean of Admissions usually chairs the committee and he or she reports directly to the Medical School Dean. The committee first evaluates students by reviewing their credentials and letters of recommendation. Committee members also conduct interviews and submit written evaluations of interviewees. The entire committee discusses each candidate's application, with the interviewer often commenting on his or her impressions. During committee meetings, all members evaluate interviewed students and participate in the voting. Meetings are usually held weekly from early fall through the end of spring.

The File

The Admissions Office maintains a file on each applicant. This file includes your AMCAS, AACOMAS, or non-AMCAS school application, your science and non-science GPA, grades from all transcripts, a list of the schools you have attended, all MCAT scores, letters of recommendation and your personal statement. In addition, your file may contain notations of support, and records of all written, verbal, and onsite inquiries you have made regarding your admission to the school.

The Personal Essay

The personal essay is the only truly personal statement you make prior to your interview. Use the essay to sell yourself. An effective essay will distinguish you from all other candidates, most of whom will have credentials nearly identical to your own. Some counsel:

Do

1. Catch the reader's attention from your first sentence. Skilled journalists know the power of a short, compelling lead. Keep your reader's attention with a well-organized, concise personal essay. A strong close will further convince your audience that it is in their best interest to interview you.

2. Describe specific accomplishments, giving the reader a well-focused and articulate view of who you are, your interests, experience and history.

3. In presenting your many achievements, do so within the context of gratitude for the opportunity rather than as a testimonial to your greatness or conquests.

4. Explain information in your application that might be viewed negatively by an admissions committee. This includes course failures, withdrawals, low MCAT scores, or other issues that might detract from your strength as an applicant.

5. Focus on honest, concrete, original, biographical information. Use your own voice. If you do quote someone, make sure the quote is highly relevant and invigorates your message. Hackneyed quotes, no; fresh, witty, wise and pertinent, yes.

6. Make your essay visually inviting to read. Revise carefully for correct punctuation, spelling and grammar. Have others critique the essay for accuracy, clarity and style.

Don't

1. Criticize your school, departments or teachers. Stay positive.

2. Discuss controversial or argumentative views. Sell yourself.

3. Try to make too many points. You have one page to convey two to three messages. Provide evidence that will convince your reader that you are a winning candidate who will make the school and the reader proud. Lead the reader to this conclusion but don't state this conclusion yourself.

Transcripts

AMCAS and AACOMAS will provide you with a Transcript Matching Form. Obtain copies of transcripts for all undergraduate schools you have attended by January of your junior year. Once you have checked these for accuracy, have the registrars send official transcripts to AMCAS, AACOMAS and non-AMCAS schools. Complete the Academic Record portion of your AMCAS, AACOMAS or non-AMCAS application and send the application. Note that the Transcript Matching Form must accompany each transcript.

Chronology

1. Request and verify accuracy of transcripts from all schools attended.
2. Have each college send official transcripts and send Transcript Matching Forms to AMCAS, AACOMAS and non-AMCAS medical schools.
3. Expect notification of receipt of transcripts from AMCAS, AACOMAS and non-AMCAS medical schools two to three weeks after requesting that these be sent.
4. Obtain AMCAS, AACOMAS and non-AMCAS application forms.
5. Complete and copy forms for your records.
6. Send completed AMCAS, AACOMAS and non-AMCAS application forms with fees.

7. Expect notification of receipt of your application from AMCAS, AACOMAS and non-AMCAS medical schools two to three weeks after you send these.

8. Pay individual medical schools' requested supplemental application fees.

9. Send mid-year grades directly to schools.

The Purpose of the Interview

The interview provides the medical school with an opportunity to learn more about applicants. It also allows the medical school to promote its own unique features. By its nature, the interview is primarily subjective. It provides useful information that actively supplements the objective information in your application.

In most cases, the interview is structured to be non-confrontational, supportive and open. Most experienced interviewers concentrate on lowering the stress level rather than raising it, and expect the applicants to be relaxed and to be themselves. Within this open setting, the applicants are provided enough time to thoughtfully answer questions.

The institution seeks women and men with outstanding intellectual and personal qualifications. The admissions committee works to select a group of individuals who are diverse in backgrounds, training and talents, yet will function well together as a class.

Interviews help the committee identify a cohesive group of highly qualified individuals.

Qualifications Evaluated

Objective (GPA, MCAT) and subjective (recommendations, personal essay, interview) criteria help the admissions committee evaluate your application. These objective and subjective tools reveal your:

1. Personality
2. Maturity and honesty
3. Interpersonal skills
4. Communication skills
5. Motivation and commitment to practice medicine
6. Leadership qualities
7. Humanistic, social, and ethical concerns
8. Depth and breadth of knowledge
9. Critical thinking and coping skills
10. Creativity and original thinking

Committee Assessment

Generally, the interviewer is asked to prepare a report as soon as possible after the interview. Most evaluations are written in the interviewer's narrative style. The interviewer is asked to create a synopsis of the interview with his or her impressions. Often, the report will include interesting highlights that have been gleaned from the application folder. Most institutions grade interviews and merge interview scores with scores for MCATs, GPA, and letters of recommendation. The summation of these four scores creates a composite score. Then, candidates are ranked as outstanding, excellent, very good, good or average.

A formal presentation of the candidate before the entire committee occurs a week or two after the interview. Objective scores of GPA, both science and nonscience, MCATs, and grades for letters of recommendation and interviews are presented to the committee. The interviewer is often asked to summarize the candidate and he or she uses this opportunity to promote the student's candidacy, reinforcing unique strengths and providing explanation for any weaknesses in the application. A full discussion ensues with questions directed to the interviewer. Finally, a consensus is reached as to whether the applicant should be accepted or denied admission.

Protocol for Tracking Status of Application

Medical schools emphasize the integrity of the admissions process. The interviewer acts as an agent of the committee, and the decision whether to admit an applicant is a committee decision. All inquiries and communications that follow your interview should be directed to the admissions office. Do not attempt to contact the interviewer or Dean of Admissions directly or through agents for yourself. The Dean of Admissions will contact you when a decision is made.

One caveat: often students withhold all communications with the admissions office for fear of "bothering them." In some medical schools, the number of oral and written contacts with the admissions office are tracked as a reflection of your interest. You should always write the Dean of Admissions and your interviewer a thank you note following your interview. You may also check the status of your application from time to time and express your continued interest in the school.

10 Common Mistakes

1. Inadequate preparation for MCAT exams
MCAT performance mirrors SAT performance. If you are an average standardized test taker, consider an MCAT review course.

2. Late application
Submit applications early. This requires excellent planning and coordination of transcripts, MCAT's, recommendations, and applications. Ideally, you should begin planning two years before you intend to enroll.

3. Poor performance in core sciences
To be competitive, A's and B's in core science

courses are generally required. An occasional C gets by, especially if accompanied by excellent MCAT's. Repeat core courses where you earned a C or below to demonstrate your mastery of the subject matter.

4. Lack of volunteer or health service experience

It has become a general expectation that candidates will pursue experiences that demonstrate growth as a caring, service-oriented individual in the field of health care. This experience exposes your understanding, and commitment to, a life of medicine.

5. Poor choice of references

A single poor reference, even subtly stated, can send an application off track. Nurture relationships with future references early. Carefully assess the level of an individual's support for you. Consider choosing those who have already demonstrated concrete support for you through grades or other forms of recognition.

6. Poor personal essay

Write a clear, concise, well-organized and interesting statement. Check its grammar, punctuation, spelling and clarity. Seek qualified or expert critique and revise accordingly.

7. Failure to monitor application status

The application process is complex and requires sequential coordinated actions. Ensure that your completed application materials are submitted and confirm their receipt by July or August.

8. Inadequate research of school

Some of the 145 medical schools will ideally suit your personality, interests and talents; others will not. Thoroughly research medical colleges by reviewing literature, visiting campuses and conferring with pre-medical advisers, alumni and current medical students. Also consider factors such as in-state versus out-of-state admission rates.

9. Inadequate preparation for your interview

Although the interview commonly carries a quarter of the decision weight, and can actually collapse an otherwise qualified applicant, many students continue to "wing it." Careful research, preparation and performance are a must. The cardinal sins: appearing arrogant or disinterested.

10. Lack of post-interview follow through

In some schools, all verbal, written and physical contacts are captured in your application file. A thank you note to the Dean of Admissions and your interviewer is always appreciated. Gratitude is a becoming attitude in everyone, and a thank you letter leaves a favorable impression on the people who may accept you. Occasional respectful contacts to check on the status of your application are generally received as an expression of continued interest.

IV
The Interview

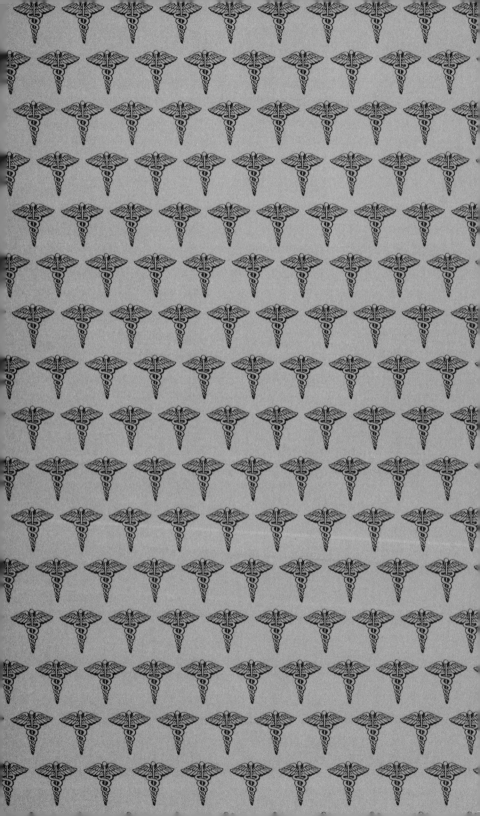

IV   The Interview

A Familiar Format

The most frequent type of interaction between two individuals is an interview with one individual soliciting information and the other providing it. Regard the medical school interview as an exchange of information. Since you were young, you have been approached and have approached others to obtain information. An interview also allows people to develop a relationship and form an impression of one other. The interview is a most flexible format that can be highly individualized. It can move forward in a prearranged manner or adapt and pursue unexpected lines of inquiry. Thorough preparation allows you to take advantage of this format. Be prepared to provide accurate and comprehensive information while keeping it positive.

Preparation for the Interview

To assure a successful interview, prepare. Think of yourself as a reporter assigned an important issue to investigate. You need a clear understanding of the organization and individuals who will be interviewing you, and the message and image you intend to convey. Review the school's catalogue and other sources of information.

1. **Conduct the following self-inventory before your interview:**
   - What is your objective?
   - What is your message and how does it support your objective?
   - Who is your audience?
   - What do you know about this institution, its people, its curriculum and its culture?
   - What do they know about you?
   - Have you reviewed your own application?
   - What within your application makes you uncomfortable?
   - What do you hope they won't ask you and how will you answer when they do?
   - Where and when is the interview?
   - Have you made adequate arrangements for lodging?
   - Have you allotted extra time so that you can arrive at your interview relaxed and on time?

2. **Interview Questions to Expect**
   Here are questions commonly asked during medical school interviews. Be prepared to answer each:
   - What do you believe in?
   - What do you care about?
   - How does that caring express itself?
   - How did you investigate a career in medicine?
   - What made you decide to pursue a career in medicine?
   - What is your favorite type of teaching style?
   - What branch of medicine most interests you?

- Who knows you the best in this world?
- How would that person describe you, and what advice have they provided you?
- What teamwork experiences have you had?
- Who are your heroes?
- What are your strengths and weaknesses?
- What skills have you developed outside the classroom?
- Where do you see yourself in 10 years?
- What is the greatest obstacle you have had to overcome?
- What issues confront medicine today? (see www.healthpolitics.com)
- What has been your greatest achievement?
- What person, past or present, would you most like to meet?
- What have you read recently in the press about health care?
- What makes you a better applicant than others?
- Why do you want to become a physician?
- How would you express your concern for a child needing an amputation?
- How do you relax?
- What is your biggest concern about entering medical school?
- Describe your best teacher and what made her or him unique.
- Describe an experience you had helping others.
- What was the last book you read?
- Describe an experience where you were misjudged.

- What has been your favorite non-science course and why?
- Who are your senators, congressional representatives, governor?
- What was your most difficult or demoralizing experience?
- What is the difference between sympathy and empathy?
- Is there anything you want to brag about or that you need to explain?
- If you are accepted to multiple schools, how will you make your decision?
- What is the toughest thing about being a patient?
- What type of criticism upsets you?
- Have you ever been a patient and, if so, can you reveal how that felt?
- How have your personal and volunteer experiences strengthened your goal to become a physician?
- What have been the strengths and weaknesses of your college preparation?
- Would you say you are most like your father or mother, and why?
- Why did you choose an osteopathic/allopathic school?
- What will you do next year if you don't get into medical school?
- Is this school your first choice?
- Why did you apply to this medical school?
- Is there anything I haven't asked you that you want to tell me?

The following subjects were covered in over two-thirds of the Class of 2009's medical school interviews:

- The source of your inspiration to pursue medicine
- Interpersonal qualities that will enhance your practice of medicine
- Specific qualities that lead to choice of this medical school
- Qualities that will insure your success as a medical school student and physician
- Interest in generalist versus specialist fields

The following topics are commonly raised regarding medical ethics:

- Privacy
- Children's rights
- Rights of the handicapped
- Rights of the terminally ill
- Rights of newborns with congenital conditions
- Organ donation
- Care of the mentally handicapped
- Care of the elderly
- Determination of death
- Physician's responsibility for societal health

3. Physical Appearance

Physical appearance creates a first impression and impacts how you are perceived. Present yourself in a personable and professional manner. Some dress for success tips:

- Dress conservatively. Men should wear a suit or a blazer and neatly pressed pants with a dress

shirt and simple tie. Women should wear a suit or
solid dress.

- Women should avoid distracting or flashy jewelry.
- Jackets should be free of lapel pins.
- Remove bulky items from pockets.
- Collar and tie should be straight. Scarves should
  be in place.
- Avoid half-glasses or light-sensitive ones that
  conceal your eyes.

4. Body Language

Physicians are expected to be skilled communica-
tors whose facial expressions and hand gestures carry
their message. Your body language is closely observed
by a physician interviewer. The following gestures
convey sincerity and interest:

- Make eye contact while you are listening.
- Sit erect but not stiff, leaning slightly forward.
- Use normal conversational hand movements to
  underscore your message.
- Listen intently to all questions and responses
  from the interviewer.

Avoid the following:

- Fidgeting or nervous gestures
- Inappropriate smiling or laughter
- Tightly grasping the arms of a chair or your
  hands in a prayer gesture
- Tightening and loosening your facial muscles
- Unnaturally straight, rigid posture
- Wandering eyes, particularly when you are
  addressed or speaking

Interview Recommendations

1. There is no consistency from one interviewer to the next. Styles and approaches vary. Expect anything.

2. Most interviews are open and non-combative. Approach the interview with optimism.

3. Honesty is key.

4. Be prepared for questions regarding weaknesses or discrepancies in your application.

5. Don't list any honors, research projects, or volunteer experiences in your application that you will be unable to support as real and significant.

6. Ask questions if you have real ones about the school.

7. Read the school catalogue prior to the interview.

8. Do not ask what your chances are.

9. Do not get upset if the interviewer is late.

10. Allow the interviewer to interrupt you, but don't interrupt the interviewer.

11. Elaborate, but don't dominate conversation.

12. Know your application file better than the interviewer (excluding your letters of recommendation).

13. Don't ask questions about your letters of recommendation if you have waived your right to see them.

14. Know something about the city you are visiting, even if only from that day's local newspaper or the taxi driver.

15. Don't try to second-guess the interviewer.

16. Avoid slang terms.

17. Be courteous and considerate toward all office staff.

18. If you know a student or faculty member personally, feel free to weave this naturally into the conversation, identifying her or him as a source of guidance and advice.

19. If this school is your first choice, state it. If not, explain your first choice if asked, and present this school as your second, if this is accurate.

20. If your choice of this school is tied to a fiancee's or spouse's choice, state it. Most schools are sympathetic to couples.

Optimal Arrival for the Interview

A thoroughly planned arrival tips the odds in your favor. If the interview is not in your immediate area, come the day before and stay overnight in a hotel or at a friend's home. Be sure that the accommodations are adequate for a good night's sleep and grooming the following morning. If possible, preview the physical site where the interview will take place. If you have the interview room number, arrive early to familiarize yourself with the location. Seeing the site with its physical arrangement avoids any sense of surprise that might shake your confidence during the interview. Awaken that morning with plenty of extra time so that you can properly groom, eat, and arrive with time to spare. Use the bathroom prior to the interview to check your clothes and your smile in the mirror.

Review the following quick tips for success:

1. Be honest

2. Be professional

3. Think fast, but speak slowly

4. Be human and interesting

5. Smile. Believe in yourself and you will transfer this belief to your interviewer.

Relaxation Techniques

Most candidates experience appropriate anxiety as they approach their interview. Remember that confidence is earned and you only acquire it by meeting challenges in a positive, determined spirit. If nervous in the final hour, try the following:

- Walk around the block, let your muscles relax, your eyes wander and b-r-e-a-t-h-e. Whistle. Sing.

- Stretch your arms, legs, torso and facial muscles.

- Think of treasured or humorous memories. Smile or laugh.

- Breathe deeply, counting for a number of seconds, then hold your breath the equivalent number of seconds and finally exhale for as long as you can. Repeat this, each time lengthening the breath, the hold and the exhalation.

- If you are in a room awaiting the interviewer's arrival, practice deep breathing and alternately tense and relax your muscles, head to toe.

- Acknowledge that even seasoned professionals experience some stage fright. If controlled, this energizes and enhances your performance.

- Remember to believe in the very best within you.

The Appearance

The interview begins when the interviewer enters the room. Rise and greet the interviewer professionally with a firm handshake and a smile. Express your pleasure and gratitude for the opportunity to interview at this medical school. While the interviewer will take the lead and ask the questions, it's important to keep in mind that you mutually own this interview. Ideally, you will enjoy an interpersonal exchange that connects and enriches you both.

Some key points:

1. Be personal and professional
Doctors may begin somewhat formally. Interviews often begin tensely and gradually yield to a warmer, more relaxed atmosphere. Mirror the mood of the interviewer and stay positive.

2. Stay on message
You should have in mind two or three points that you wish to convey during the interview. Seek opportunities early to introduce and reinforce these points.

3. Practice active listening
Listen carefully to questions posed. Clarify any inquiry or information that is unclear before you respond.

4. Control the pace
When nervous, most people speak too quickly. A controlled, slower pace shows a contemplative, more self-possessed candidate.

5. Monitor your body language
Be aware that your body is a powerful communication tool.

6. Stay alert, polite, poised

Skilled interviewers will attempt to relax you so that you will be honest and spontaneous with them. Their goal is to get to know the real you. This is your goal as well. Remember, though, that you need to maintain a polished, professional demeanor.

7. Maintain respectful, interested eye contact

Use eye contact as you would when fully engaged in an interesting conversation with a friend.

8. Affirm the positive

If asked a question that provides an opportunity to voice something you think is important, restate the question during your response. You might even reveal that you are glad the interviewer broached the subject.

9. Proceed mindfully

Stay within the bounds of a professional interview. The interviewer is not a trusted confidante or close friend. Rather, the interviewer is appraising your personal qualities and communication skills. Humor can jeopardize your candidacy. You needn't be stiff or refrain from smiling. Just save your favorite joke for a more appropriate audience.

10. Enjoy the interview and learn from it

At the end of your meeting, you will know more about the interviewer, yourself, and this prospective medical school. Your performance will be improved by an attitude that emphasizes exploration rather than fear.

Tough Questions...

Foresee tough questions or those that come from left field. Try to provide a reasonable and informed response. It is not so much what you say, but how you say it. Some counsel:

1. Acknowledge that this is a difficult question. This shows that you are listening and gives you a few moments to prepare a reasoned, balanced response.

2. Demonstrate concern and thoughtfulness in your response and maintain a moderate voice.

3. Above all, don't take a tough question personally. Often, an interviewer poses difficult questions to test your resilience.

4. Do not argue or become defensive. The last thing you want to do is dispute the interviewer.

5. Modulate your body language. You may want to verbally retaliate, but your body should do just the opposite. This softens the impact of the trying question and demonstrates your equilibrium.

6. Segue to a more favorable message. While addressing the question, relate it to a subject that contains some of the major messages you want to convey. Candidates who can turn the tables diplomatically prove their mettle and grace.

7. Don't be overwhelmed. Your whole life is not on the line. If one hard question can undo you, you may not be able to withstand the rigors of this demanding profession.

8. Conclude your response on an amicable, positive note.

Post Interview Self-Evaluation

Now that you have made it through the interview, your work isn't over. Breathe, walk, eat, and then sit down within an hour of your interview and answer the following questions:

1. Did I stay on message?

2. Was I in control?

3. Did I tell the truth and avoid exaggeration?

4. Was I calm and did I pace myself well?

5. Did I anticipate the questions?

6. Did I present a positive, professional image?

7. Did I listen carefully?

8. Was I a credible candidate?

9. Could I have done better and how?

10. What did I learn?

There's always something you could have done a little bit better. Through conscientious introspection, you will continually develop your interpersonal skills.

Summary of Interview Advice

In summation:

1. Be Prepared: Have something to say. Say it with style, force and intelligence.

2. Be Human: Medicine requires excellent communication and people skills, composure and poise. During your interview, demonstrate your maturity, thoughtfulness and sensitivity.

3. Be Yourself: Physicians regularly practice reading people's overt and covert responses. Be yourself, trust in your preparation and in human nature and learn from your experience.

Good luck!

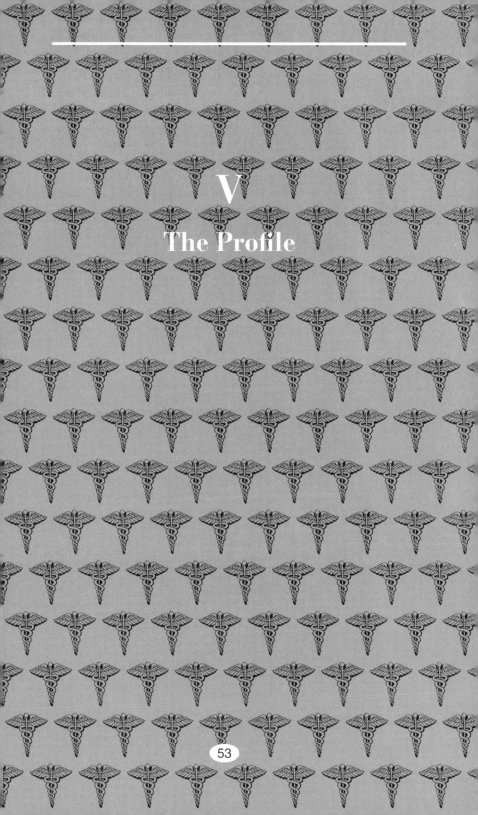

V
The Profile

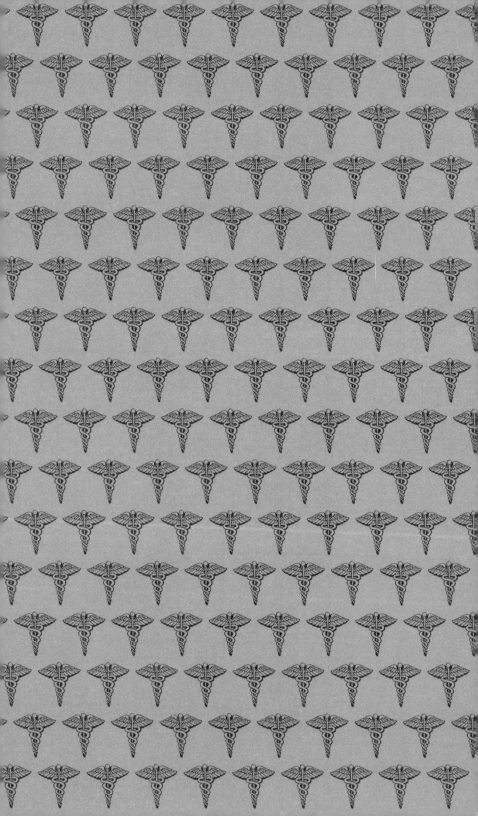

V The Profile

Allopathic: Class of 2009 (entering Fall 2005)
- 125 allopathic schools
- 37,364 applicants
  - 49.8% women
  - 50.2% men
- 17,978 acceptance offered
- 17,004 entrants
  - 48.5% women
  - 51.5% men
- 14% Black and Hispanic entrants

Average Entrant Scores

MCAT
VR	9.7
PS	10.1
BS	10.4

GPA
Sciences	3.56
Total	3.63

Osteopathic: Class of 2009 (entering Fall 2005)
- 22 osteopathic schools (three branch campuses)
- 9,736 applicants
- 3,880 entrants
- 39% acceptance
- 50% women
- 8% Black and Hispanic entrants

Average Entrant Scores

MCAT
VR	8.31
PS	8.04
BS	8.64

GPA
Sciences	3.35
Total	3.45

Medical Students' Beliefs:

A 2005 survey of matriculating medical students conducted by the Association of American Medical Colleges revealed the following beliefs:

1. Everyone is entitled to receive adequate medical care regardless of his ability to pay.

2. Physicians' legal liabilities and the high cost of malpractice insurance are major problems.

3. Access to medical care continues to be a major problem in the United States.

4. Physicians have an opportunity to exercise greater influence on health promotion and disease.

5. Physicians have an obligation to care for a reasonable number of patients who will be unable to pay for the services they receive.

6. Advances in the biomedical sciences and their application to the care of patients will make the practice of medicine more challenging and rewarding in the near future.

7. Use of animals in research is necessary for the advancement of medicine.

8. Having interesting and intelligent colleagues is a major benefit of being a physician.

9. Changes in the healthcare system are impairing physician's independence.

10. Relief of patients' suffering is the most important pursuit of medicine.

Top five reasons for choosing medicine:

1. Profession provides opportunity to make a difference in people's lives.

2. Physicians can educate patients about health promotion and disease prevention.

3. Profession provides opportunity to exercise social responsibility.

4. Physicians use critical thinking to evaluate medical findings.

5. Being a physician is one of the most intellectually challenging professions.

Top five reasons students chose a particular medical school:

1. Geographic location.

2. Friendliness of the administrator, faculty, and/or students.

3. Teaching methods of school.

4. Ability of school to place students in paraticularly residency programs.

5. Nature of school's curriculum.

CLASS OF 2009

Medical School	Class Size	% In-State Pupils	% Women	Resident Tuition	Non-Resident Tuition
Alabama					
University of Alabama*	160	90	44	11,365	34,095
University of South Alabama*	68	87	44	12,254	24,508
Arizona					
Arizona COM §	163	27	46	38,908	38,908
University of Arizona	110	99	51	14,359	N/A
Arkansas					
University of Arkansas	148	94	46	12,806	25,612
California					
University of California Davis*	93	96	47	0	12,245
University of California Irvine*	103	98	46	0	12,245
University of California Los Angeles*	170	84	60	0	12,245
University of California San Diego*	121	92	44	0	12,245
University of California San Francisco*	153	82	60	0	12,245
Loma Linda University	171	48	44	31,692	31,692
KECK School of Medicine of the University of Southern California	171	73	48	39,198	39,198
Stanford University	85	36	48	38,925	38,925
Touro University COM §	135	40	60	34,110	34,110
Western University of the Health Sciences* §	216	70	49	37,190	37,190
Colorado					
University of Colorado	143	76	51	20,713	72,291
Connecticut					
University of Connecticut*	79	75	71	15,870	36,110
Yale University	100	9	58	37,280	37,280

CLASS OF 2009

Medical School	Class Size	% In-State Pupils	% Women	Resident Tuition	Non-Resident Tuition
Washington, DC					
George Washington University	177	.016	56	41,193	41,193
Georgetown University	190	.015	96	37,121	37,121
Howard University	116	.008	51	22,695	22,695
Florida					
Nova Southeastern University [§]	246	57	52	35,673	35,673
Florida State University	80	100	63	17,555	47,059
University of Florida	128	96	58	18,016	45,052
University of Miami	182	82	49	29,298	38,504
University of South Florida*	120	94	52	16,449	47,005
Georgia					
Emory University	113	31	48	36,000	36,000
Medical College of Georgia	180	99	43	11,850	30,976
Mercer University	60	100	42	30,220	N/A
Morehouse School of Medicine*	52	57	59	24,000	24,000
Hawaii					
University of Hawaii	60	85	53	16,272	29,784
Illinois					
Chicago COM [§]	177	37	55	36,391	40,492
University of Chicago – The Pritzker School of Medicine	104	37	46	32,022	32,022
Rosalind Franklin University of Medicine and Science/ Chicago Medical School	185	21	49	36,740	36,740
University of Illinois	333	74	48	22,122	52,176
Loyola University – Chicago	140	46	49	34,500	34,500
Northwestern University	171	26	49	37,208	37,208
Rush Medical College	128	83	49	39,024	39,024
Southern Illinois University	72	100	53	18,312	54,936
Indiana					
Indiana University	280	85	44	20,864	40,549

CLASS OF 2009

Medical School	Class Size	% In-State Pupils	% Women	Resident Tuition	Non-Resident Tuition
Iowa					
University of Iowa	142	68	43	19,020	38,226
Des Moines University of Osteopathic Medicine and Surgery* §	216	20	49	31,720	31,720
Kansas					
University of Kansas	175	81	45	18,919	34,674
Kentucky					
University of Kentucky	103	72	45	18,342	37,316
University of Louisville	149	81	40	18,040	40,406
Pikeville College School of Osteopathic Medicine (PCSOM) §	80	44	48	N/A	N/A
Louisiana					
Louisiana State–New Orleans*	178	97	42	0	0
Louisiana State–Shreveport	108	99	44	9,776	23,924
Tulane University	155	27	48	38,172	38,172
Maine					
University of New England COM §	125	17	57	36,740	36,740
Maryland					
Johns Hopkins University*	121	.09	43	32,200	32,200
University of Maryland*	150	82	58	19,277	34,144
Uniformed Service University	169	.02	28	0	0
Massachusetts					
Boston University	155	15	59	39,510	39,510
Harvard Medical School	165	15	51	35,800	35,800
University of Massachusetts*	102	98	59	8,352	N/A
Tufts University	168	36	46	43,014	43,014

CLASS OF 2009

Medical School	Class Size	% In-State Pupils	% Women	Resident Tuition	Non-Resident Tuition
Michigan					
Michigan State University COM[§]	205	92	53	23,820	53,820
Michigan State University	106	76	58	22,377	50,277
University of Michigan	177	44	49	21,578	33,980
Wayne State University	260	89	49	21,695	45,147
Minnesota					
Mayo Clinic College of Medicine Medical School	43	26	49	24,500	24,500
University of Minnesota	220	76	47	26,607	33,502
Mississippi					
University of Mississippi	105	100	31	7,649	14,327
Missouri					
A.T. Still University of Health Sciences/Kirksville COM[§]	169	—	38	35,320	35,320
Kansas City University of Medicine and Biosciences[§]	248	13	50	36,460	36,460
University of Missouri –Columbia	96	86	55	20,909	41,634
University of Missouri –Kansas City	95	66	59	26,817	52,060
St. Louis University	153	31	40	36,960	36,960
Washington University	123	.05	51	39,720	39,720
Nebraska					
Creighton University	125	14	46	37,519	37,519
University of Nebraska	117	85	44	19,568	45,888
Nevada					
University of Nevada	52	81	50	10,588	29,398

CLASS OF 2009

Medical School	Class Size	% In-State Pupils	% Women	Resident Tuition	Non-Resident Tuition
New Hampshire					
Dartmouth Medical School	82	.09	50	34,500	34,500
New Jersey					
University of Medicine and Dentristy of NJ	170	84	49	21,390	33,472
UMDNJ –Robert Wood Johnson	157	83	50	21,390	33,472
UMDNJ–School of OM [§]	102	98	59	22,246	34,811
New Mexico					
University of New Mexico	75	93	53	12,893	37,032
New York					
Albany Medical College	135	44	63	39,637	39,637
Albert Einstein College of Medicine	180	44	57	37,550	37,550
Columbia University*	149	20	48	38,720	38,720
Cornell University Weill Medical College	101	34	50	32,320	32,320
Mt. Sinai School of Medicine	123	43	46	33,250	33,250
New York COM [§]	321	63	49	34,984	34,984
New York Medical College	186	30	51	37,200	37,200
New York University*	160	41	46	30,625	30,625
University of Rochester*	100	37	55	34,450	34,450
State University of NY –Downstate	187	87	50	18,800	33,500
University of Buffalo	140	84	60	18,800	33,500
State University of NY –Upstate (Syracuse)	120	78	58	18,800	33,500
Stony Brook University	101	91	48	16,800	29,900

CLASS OF 2009

Medical School	Class Size	% In-State Pupils	% Women	Resident Tuition	Non-Resident Tuition
North Carolina					
Duke University*	101	16	48	34,842	34,842
The Brody School of Medicine at East Carolina University	72	100	51	6,034	31,024
University of NC Chapel Hill	160	88	51	9,335	33,001
Wake Forrest University School of Medicine	109	41	41	34,006	34,006
North Dakota					
University of North Dakota	62	72	62	18,908	50,482
Ohio					
Case Western Reserve	167	26	50	37,944	37,944
University of Cincinnati	160	75	45	22,452	39,876
Medical University of Ohio	147	65	37	19,350	47,610
Northeastern Ohio University	120	95	47	33,307	46,614
Ohio State University	210	57	33	22,833	35,664
Ohio University COM [§]	115	83	57	21,858	21,858
Wright State University	100	90	57	20,988	29,712
Oklahoma					
Oklahoma State University COM [§]	93	93	48	16,045	31,265
University of Oklahoma	152	89	40	15,140	37,228
Oregon					
Oregon Health Sciences*	112	61	52	24,100	34,101
Pennsylvania					
Lake Erie COM [§]	230	28	46	N/A	N/A
Jefferson Medical College	254	42	48	38,316	38,316
Drexel University COM [§]	231	27	52	36,770	36,770
Pennsylvania State University	135	42	50	29,280	40,706
Philadelphia COM [§]	273	57	51	34,773	34,773
University of Pennsylvania	147	25	51	36,976	36,976
University of Pittsburgh	148	16	48	32,218	36,965
Temple University	176	53	47	33,730	41,310

CLASS OF 2009

Medical School	Class Size	% In-State Pupils	% Women	Resident Tuition	Non-Resident Tuition
Puerto Rico					
Universidad Central del Caribe*	63	79	51	20,000	27,000
Ponce School of Medicine	66	56	47	17,836	26,590
University of Puerto Rico	115	100	50	6,650	13,965
Rhode Island					
Brown University	73	12	58	34,472	34,472
South Carolina					
Medical University of South Carolina*	142	94	46	6,049	19,437
University of South Carolina	80	89	56	19,520	56,446
South Dakota					
University of South Dakota*	50	96	52	13,324	31,700
Tennessee					
East Tennessee State University	60	82	53	17,462	35,594
Meharry Medical College*	85	2	55	27,143	27,143
University of Tennessee	150	94	38	17,522	34,406
Vanderbilt University	105	13	48	33,200	33,200
Texas					
Baylor College of Medicine*	168	75	45	7,550	20,850
Texas A&M	83	89	53	7,550	20,850
Texas COM §	140	96	50	10,150	25,900
Texas Tech University	140	95	46	8,550	21,650
University of Texas–Dallas	229	83	45	9,325	22,245
University of Texas –Galveston*	210	94	51	8,350	21,450
University of Texas –Houston	210	97	47	9,775	22,875
University of Texas –San Antonio*	206	96	52	9,550	23,725

CLASS OF 2009

Medical School	Class Size	% In-State Pupils	% Women	Resident Tuition	Non-Resident Tuition
Utah					
University of Utah	102	73	38	16,973	32,133
Vermont					
University of Vermont	101	42	57	24,000	42,010
Virginia					
Eastern Virginia Medical School	110	66	53	20,521	37,933
Edward Via Virginia COM §	160	29	48	29,995	29,995
Virginia Commonwealth University	184	56	48	22,385	36,414
University of Virginia	141	65	46	27,073	36,897
Washington					
University of Washington	180	91	47	13,952	33,790
West Virginia					
Marshall University	60	82	43	14,610	38,000
West Virginia School of Osteopathic Medicine §	111	49	43	18,886	46,736
West Virginia University School of Medicine	98	58	35	14,766	34,254
Wisconsin					
Medical College of Wisconsin	204	47	45	28,503	33,370
University of Wisconsin	163	82	53	21,202	32,326

* The tuition figures above do not include student fees. Student fees range from $500 to $1,500 for most schools. Schools marked with an asterisk have student fees ranging from $2,500 to $7,000.

Contact schools directly to confirm current student tuition and fees.

§ Denotes osteopathic medical school.

N/A Denotes not applicable.

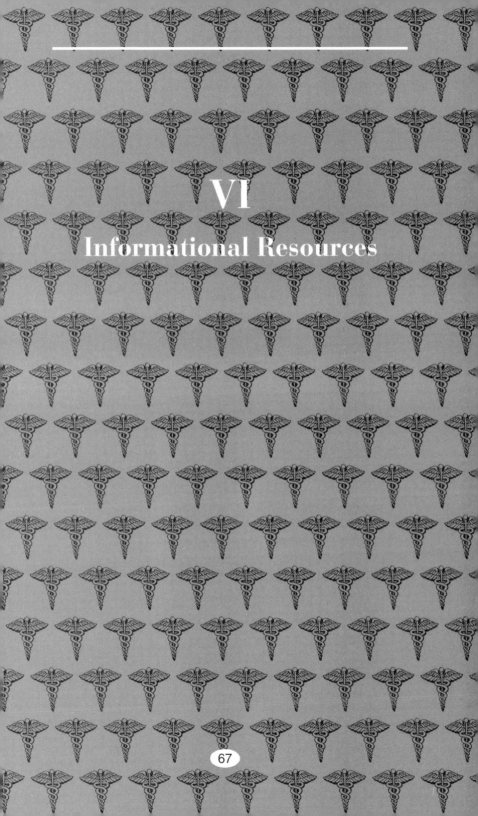

VI
Informational Resources

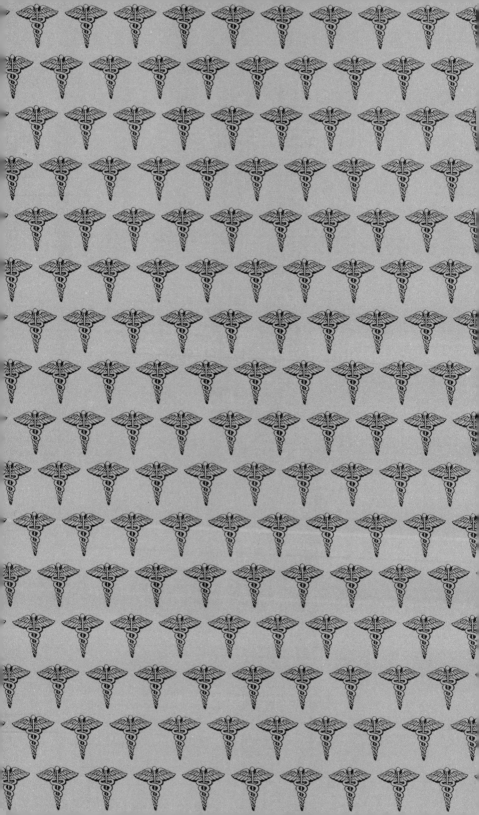

VI Informational Resources

Print Information

These printed resources may be useful supplements to your educational and financial planning:

1. *Funding Education Beyond High School, 2006-2007.* Department of Education. Free. EDPubs. P.O. Box 1398, Jessup, M.D. 20794-1398, (877) 433-7827; www.edpubs.org

2. *The Book of Majors* , 2007. Item #007654. $24.95, plus sales tax where applicable. Revised annually. College Board Publications, P.O. Box 869010, Plano, TX 75074; 800-323-7155; www.collegeboard.com

3. *Need a Lift? College Financial Aid Handbook, 2007.* Item #755.507. $3.00 prepaid, plus sales tax where applicable and shipping and handling. The American Legion Emblem Sales, P.O. Box 1050, Indianapolis, IN 46206; (888) 453-4466

4. *Medical School Admission Requirements United States and Canada 2007-2008.* $25.00 plus shipping. Association of American Medical Colleges, 2450 N Street, NW, Washington, DC 20037; (202) 828-0416; www.aamc.org

5. *Health Professions Career & Education Directory, 2006-2007 edition.* $70.00, non-members; $52.50 members, plus shipping and handling. Order No. OP-417506. American Medical Association. To order call (800) 621-8335.

6. *300 Ways To Put Your Talent To Work in the Health Field.* $18.00, non-members; $15.00, members, plus $5.00 shipping and handling. National Health Council, 1730 M Street, NW, Suite 500, Washington, DC 20036; (202) 785-3910; go to www.nationalhealthcouncil.org to order.

7. *Essays That Will Get You into Medical School.* 2nd Edition, By Dan Kaufman, Chris Dowhan, Adrienne Dowhan, $12.95 paperback, Barrons Educational Series, Inc., 250 Wireless Blvd, Hauppauge NY, 11788; 1-800-645-3476

8. *The Pact.* By Rameck Hunt, Samson Davis, Lisa Page, George Jenkins,. $14.00 paperback, Riverhead Books, Penguin Group (USA) Inc., 405 Murray Hill Parkway, East Rutherford, NJ 07073; 1-800-788-6262

9. *The Best Medicine.* By Mike Magee, Michael D'Antonio, $23.95, Spencer Books, New York, NY, www.spencerbooks.com; 1-866-543-5140

10. *Health Politics: Power, Populism and Health.* By Mike Magee, $39.95, Spencer Books, New York, NY; to order, call 1-866-543-5140

Health Careers Information

These professional associations provide information useful to health professionals:

1. Association of American Medical Colleges
   2450 N Street, NW
   Washington, DC 20037
   (202) 828-0400
   www.aamc.org

2. American Association of Colleges of Osteopathic Medicine
   Suite 310
   5550 Friendship Boulevard
   Chevy Chase, MD 20815-7231
   (301) 968-4100
   www.aacom.org

3. American Association of Colleges of Pharmacy
   1426 Prince Street
   Alexandria, VA 22314-2841
   (703) 739-2330
   www.aacp.org

4. American Association of Colleges of Podiatric Medicine
   Suite 320
   1580 Crabbs Branch Way
   Rockville, MD 20855
   (800) 922-9266
   www.aacpm.org

5. American Dental Education Association
   Suite 1100
   1400 K Street, NW
   Washington, DC 20005
   (202) 289-7201
   www.adea.org

6. Association of American Veterinary Medical Colleges
   Suite 301
   1101 Vermont Avenue, NW
   Washington, DC 20005
   (202) 371-9195
   www.aavmc.org

7. Association of Schools and Colleges of Optometry
   Suite 510
   6110 Executive Boulevard
   Rockville, MD 20852
   (301) 231-5944
   www.opted.org

8. Association of Schools of Public Health
   1101 15th Street, NW
   Suite 910
   Washington, DC 20005
   (202) 296-1099
   www.asph.org

9. National Association of Advisors for the Health Professions
   P.O. Box 1518
   Champaign, IL 61824-1518
   (217) 355-0063
   www.naahp.org

10. Alpha Epsilon Delta
    National Office
    James Madison University
    MSC 9015
    Blue #309
    601 University Blvd.
    Harrisonburg, VA 22807
    (540) 568-2594
    www.jmu.edu/orgs/nationalaed

Electronic Information:

www.healthpolitics.com – a weekly, Internet-based electronic media program that explores complex topics at the intersection of health-care and policy.

www.positiveprofiles.com – Pfizer Medical Humanities Initiative; offers email access to medical schools nationwide, publications, scholarship information, physician profiles, inspirational stories, links to other resources.

www.aamc.org – offers information on America's 125 allopathic medical schools.

www.aamc.org/students/financing/md2/start.htm – (MD)2 : Monetary Decisions for Medical Doctors is a comprehensive, three-part program developed by the AAMC to assist premedical and medical students in their planning for the financial aspects of their medical education.

www.services.aamc.org/postbac/ – AAMC's database of postbaccalaurate premedical programs.

www.aacom.org – offers information on America's 20 osteopathic medical schools.

www.ama-assn.org/go/becominganmd – offers information on becoming an M.D.

www.ama-assn.org/ama/pub/category/2322.html – offers information on careers in allied health professions.

www.kaplan.com – offers MCAT preparation and information.

www.review.com – offers MCAT preparation and information.

www.naahp.org – National Association of Advisors for the Health Professions

www.asph.org – Association of Schools of Public Health

www.jmu.edu/orgs/nationalaed – national medical honor society, Alpha Epsilon Delta

www.aacp.org – American Association of Colleges of Pharmacy

www.aacpm.org – American Association of Colleges of Podiatric Medicine

www.adea.org – American Dental Education Association

www.aavmc.org – Association of American Veterinary Medical Colleges

www.opted.org – Association of Schools and Colleges of Optometry

Medical Science Information:

www.ama-assn.org – The American Medical Association

www.cmwf.org – The Commonwealth Fund

www.drkoop.com – Dr. Koop

www.healthpolitics.com

www.jama.ama-assn.org – The Journal of the American Medical Association

www.mayohealth.org – Mayo Clinic Health Oasis

www.nhionline.net – National Health Information

www.nih.gov – National Institutes of Health

www.nejm.org – The New England Journal of Medicine

www.pfizer.com – Pfizer Inc

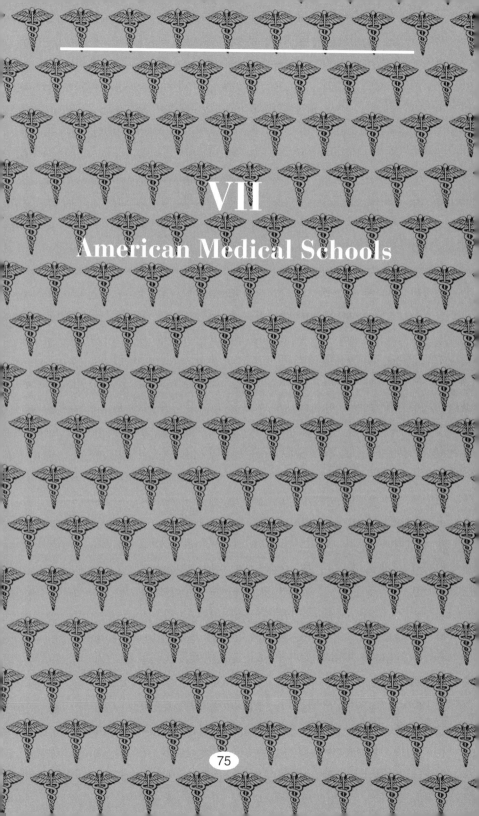

VII

American Medical Schools

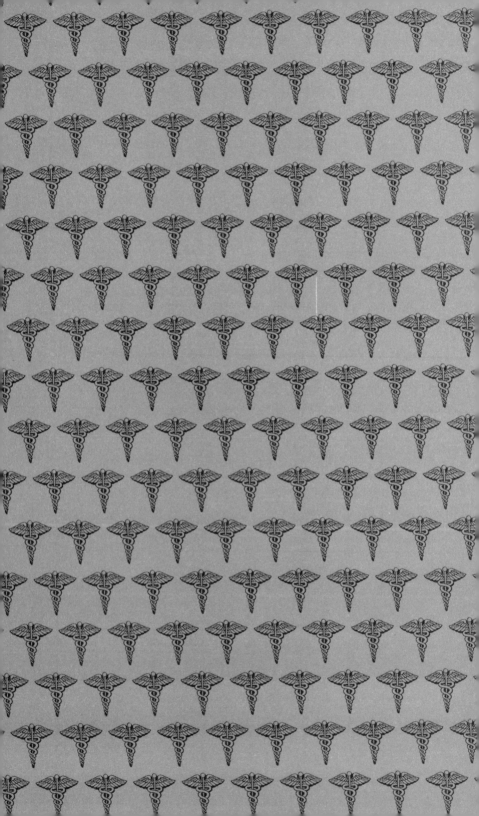

VII American Medical Schools

Admissions Contact Person & Address

ALABAMA

University of Alabama
School of Medicine
Dr. Nathan Smith
Assistant Dean for Admissions
Office of Medical Student
Services/Admissions VH-100
1530 3rd Avenue South
Birmingham, AL 35294-0019
205-934-2333

University of South Alabama
College of Medicine
Mark Scott
Director for Admissions
Office of Admissions 241 CSAB
Mobile, AL 36688-0002
251-460-7176

ARIZONA

Arizona College of Osteopathic
Medicine [§]
Jim Walter
Director of Admissions
19555 N. 59th Avenue
Glendale, AZ 85308
888-247-9277

A.T. Still University College of
Osteopathic Medicine—Mesa [§]
Joyce Haynie
Associate Director of Arizona
Admissions
5850 E. Still Circle
Mesa, AZ 85206
866-626-2870 ext. 2237

University of Arizona
College of Medicine
Dr. Christopher Leadem
Senior Associate Dean for
Admissions and Student Affairs
Admissions Office
P.O. Box 245075
Tucson, AZ 85724-5075
520-626-6214

ARKANSAS

University of Arkansas for Medical
Sciences College of Medicine
Tom G. South
Director of Student Admissions
and Financial Aid
4301 W. Markham St., Slot 551
Little Rock, AR 72205-7199
501-686-5354

CALIFORNIA

University of California–
Davis School of Medicine
Dr. Edward Dagang
Director of Admissions and
Outreach Admissions
Admissions Office
1 Shield Avenue
Davis, CA 95616
530-752-2717

University of California–
Irvine School of Medicine
Gayle Pierce
Director of Admissions
Office of Admissions and Outreach
Berk Hall, Room 100
Irvine, CA 92697-4089
800-824-5388

University of California–Los Angeles
   David Gefton at UCLA School
   of Medicine
Dr. Neil Parker
Dean for Admissions and Students
P.O. Box 957035
Office of Student Affairs
159 Center for Health Sciences
Los Angeles, CA 90095
310-825-6081

University of California–San Diego
   School of Medicine
Dr. Carolyn Kelly
Associate Dean for Admissions and
   Students
UCSDSOM Admission
0621/Medical Teaching Facility
9500 Gilman Drive
LaJolla, CA 92093-0621
858-534-3880

University of California–
   San Francisco
   School of Medicine
Dr. David Wofsy
Associate Dean of Admissions
C-200, Box 0408
San Francisco, CA 94143-0408
415-476-4044

Loma Linda University
   School of Medicine
Stephen Nyirady, Ph.D.
Associate Dean for Admissions
Loma Linda, CA 92350
909-558-4467

KECK School of Medicine of the
University of Southern California
Dr. Erin Quinn
Associate Dean of Admissions
1975 Zonal Avenue (KAM 100-C)
Los Angeles, CA 90089-9021
323-442-2552

Stanford University
   School of Medicine
Dr. Gabriel Garcia
Associate Dean for Medical School
   Admissions
251 Campus Drive
MSOB Room X3C01
Stanford, CA 94305-5404
650-723-6861

Touro University
   College of Osteopathic Medicine [§]
Dr. Donald Haight
Director of Admissions
1310 Johnson Lane
Vallejo, CA 94592
888-887-7336

Western University of the Health
   Sciences/College of Osteopathic
   Medicine of the Pacific [§]
Susan Hanson
Director of Admissions
309 East 2nd Street
Pomona, CA 91766-1854
909-469-5335

COLORADO

University of Colorado
   School of Medicine
Dr. Henry Sondheimer
Associate Dean for Admissions
4200 E. Ninth Avenue, C-297
Denver, CO 80262
303-315-7361

CONNECTICUT

University of Connecticut
   School of Medicine
Keat Sanford, Ph.D.
Assistant Dean for Admissions
263 Farmington Ave., Rm AG-062
Farmington, CT 06030-3906
860-679-4713

78

Yale University
   School of Medicine
Dr. Thomas L. Lentz
Associate Dean – Admissions and
Financial Aid
Office of Admissions
367 Cedar Street
New Haven, CT 06510
203-785-2643

WASHINGTON, DC

George Washington University
   School of Medicine and Health
   Sciences
Dianne McQuail
Assistant Dean for Admissions
Ross Hall 716
2300 I Street, NW, Room 716
Washington, DC 20037
202-994-3506

Georgetown University
   School of Medicine
Eugene T. Ford
Assistant Dean for Admissions
Office of Admissions
Box 571421
Washington, DC 20057
202-687-1154

Howard University
   College of Medicine
Ann Finney
Admissions Officer
520 W Street, NW
Washington, DC 20059
202-806-6270

FLORIDA

Nova Southeastern University
   College of Osteopathic Medicine [S]
Marla Frohlinger
Executive Director of Student
   Services and Professional
   Coordination
3200 S. University Drive
Fort Lauderdale, FL 33328
954-262-1101

Florida State University
   College of Medicine
Dr. Peter Eveland
Associate Dean of Student Affairs,
   Admissions and Outreach
Administration Building,
Room 1110-F
Tallahassee, FL 32306-4300
850-644-7904

University of Florida
   College of Medicine
Robyn Sheppard
Director of Admissions
P.O. Box 100216
UF Health Sciences Center
Gainesville, FL 32610
352-392-4569

University of Miami
   School of Medicine
Dr. R.E. Hinkley
Associate Dean for Admissions and
   Enrollment Management
P.O. Box 016159
Miami, FL 33101
305-243-6791

University of South Florida
   College of Medicine
Dr. Steve Specter
Associate Dean for Admissions and
   Student Affairs
12901 Bruce B. Downs Blvd.
MDC3
Tampa, FL 33612-4799
813-974-2229

GEORGIA

Emory University
 School of Medicine
Dr. J. William Eley, Executive
Associate Dean for Medical
 Education / Student Affairs
Woodruff Health Sciences Building
1440 Clifton Road, NE, Room 115
Atlanta, GA 30322-4510
404-727-5660

Medical College of Georgia
 School of Medicine
Dr. Mason Thompson
Associate Dean for Admissions
Augusta, GA 30912-4760
706-721-3186

Mercer University
 School of Medicine
Dr. Roger W. Comeau
Associate Dean for Admissions
Office of Admissions, & Student
 Affairs, Minority Affairs
1550 College Street
Macon, GA 31207
478-301-2542

Morehouse School of Medicine
Dr. Angela Franklin
Vice Dean for Academic and
 Student Affairs
720 Westview Drive, SW
Atlanta, GA 30310-1495
404-752-1650

HAWAII

University of Hawaii
John A. Burns School of Medicine
Dr. Satoru Izutsu
Senior Associate Dean
651 Ilalo Street
Honolulu, HI 96813
808-692-1000

ILLINOIS

Chicago College of Osteopathic
 Medicine [S]
Michael Laken
Director of Admissions
555 31st Street
Downer's Grove, IL 60515
630-515-7200

University of Chicago
 Division of the Biological Sciences
 The Pritzker School of Medicine
Sylvia Robertson
Assistant Dean of Admissions and
 Financial Aid
924 E. 57th Street, BSLC 104W
Chicago, IL 60637-5416
773-702-1937

Rosalind Franklin University
 of Medicine and Science
 Chicago Medical School
Maryann De Caire
Executive Director of Admissions,
 Records and Financial Aid
3333 Green Bay Road
N. Chicago, IL 60064
847-578-3204

University of Illinois
 College of Medicine
Dr. Jorge A. Girotti
Associate Dean and Director
808 S. Wood Street
Room 165 CME M/C 783
Chicago, IL 60612-7302
312-996-5635

Loyola University Chicago
 Stritch School of Medicine
LaDonna E. Norstrom
Assistant Dean, Admissions
Office of Admissions
2160 S. First Avenue
Maywood, IL 60153
708-216-3229

Northwestern University
 Feinberg School of Medicine
Dolores Brown
Associate Dean for Admissions
303 E. Chicago Avenue
Morton 1-606
Chicago, IL 60611-3008
312-503-8206

Rush Medical College of Rush
 University
Jan L. Schmidt
Director of Admissions
524 Armour Academic Center
600 S. Paulina Street
Suite 524
Chicago, IL 60612
312-942-6913

Southern Illinois University
 School of Medicine
Evan Wilson
Director of Admissions
Office of Student Admissions
P.O. Box 19624
Springfield, IL 62794-9624
217-545-6013

INDIANA

Indiana University
 School of Medicine
Mr. Robert M. Stump, Jr.
Director of Admissions
Fesler Hall 213
1120 South Drive
Indianapolis, IN 46202-5113
317-274-3772

IOWA

University of Iowa
 Roy J. and Lucille A. Carver
 College of Medicine
Catherine Solow
Assistant Dean, Student Affairs
100 Medicine Administration
 Building
Iowa City, IA 52242-1101
319-335-8052

Des Moines University
 College of Osteopathic Medicine [§]
Margie Gehringer
Director of Admissions &
 Enrollment Development
3200 Grand Avenue
Des Moines, IA 50312
515-271-1499

KANSAS

University of Kansas
 School of Medicine
Sandra J. McCurdy, M.Ed.
Associate Dean for Admissions
Mail Stop 1049
3901 Rainbow Boulevard
Kansas City, KS 66160
913-588-5245

KENTUCKY

University of Kentucky
 College of Medicine
Dr. Carol L. Elam
Assistant Dean for Admissions
Admissions Room MN-118
Office of Medical Education
800 Rose Street
Lexington, KY 40536-0298
859-323-6161

University of Louisville
School of Medicine
Dr. Stephen F. Wheeler
Associate Dean, Medical School
Admissions
Abell Administration Center
323 East Chestnut Street
Louisville, KY 40202-3866
502-852-5193

Pikeville College
School of Osteopathic Medicine
(PCSOM) [§]
Angel Hamilton
Director of Admissions
147 Sycamore Street
Pikeville, KY 41501
606-218-5406

LOUISIANA

Louisiana State University
School of Medicine in
New Orleans
Dr. Sam G. McClugage, Jr.
Associate Dean for Admissions
1901 Perdido Street, Box P3-4
New Orleans, LA 70112-1393
504-568-6262

Louisiana State University Health
Sciences Center
School of Medicine in Shreveport
Dr. F. Scott Kennedy
Assistant Dean for Student
Admissions
P.O. Box 33932
Shreveport, LA 71130-3932
318-675-5190

Tulane University
School of Medicine
Dr. Marc J. Kahn
Associate Dean for Admissions and
Student Affairs
1430 Tulane Avenue, SL67
New Orleans, LA 70112-2699
504-588-5187

MAINE

University of New England
College Osteopathic Medicine [§]
Lisa Lane
Asst. Director Medical Admissions
11 Hills Beach Road
Biddeford, ME 04005
207-283-0171, ext. 2218

MARYLAND

Johns Hopkins University
School of Medicine
Dr. James Weiss
Associate Dean for Admissions
733 North Broadway, Suite G-49
Baltimore, MD 21205
410-955-3182

University of Maryland
School of Medicine
Dr. Milford M. Foxwell, Jr.
Associate Dean for Admissions
655 W. Baltimore St.
Baltimore, MD 21201-1599
410-706-7478

Uniformed Services University of
the Health Sciences
F. Edward Hébert School of
Medicine
Peter J. Stavish, L.T.C, M.S., U.S.A. (Ret)
Assistant Dean for Admissions &
Academic Records
Admissions Office, Room A-1041
4301 Jones Bridge Road
Bethesda, MD 20814-4799
301-295-3101

MASSACHUSETTS

Boston University
  School of Medicine
Dr. Robert Witzburg
Associate Dean and Director of
  Admissions
Building L, Room 124
715 Albany Street
Boston, MA 02118
617-638-4630

Harvard Medical School
Robert J. Mayer, M.D.
Faculty Associate Dean for
  Admissions
25 Shattuck Street
Boston, MA 02115-6092
617-432-1550

University of Massachusetts
  Medical School
Dr. Jon Paraskos
Associate Dean for Admissions
55 Lake Avenue, N, Room 51-112
Worcester, MA 01655
508-856-2323

Tufts University
  School of Medicine
Thomas M. Slavin
Director of Admissions
136 Harrison Avenue
Boston, MA 02111
617-636-6571

MICHIGAN

Michigan State University
  College of Osteopathic Medicine [§]
Kathie Schaefer
Director of Admissions
A136 East Fee Hall
East Lansing, MI 48824-1316
517-353-7740

Michigan State University
  College of Human Medicine
Christine L. Shafer, M.D.
Asst. Dean, Admissions
A-239 Life Sciences
East Lansing, MI 48824-1317
517-353-9620

University of Michigan
  Medical School
Dr. Daniel Remick
Assistant Dean, Admissions
4303, Medical Science Building I
Ann Arbor, MI 48109-0624
734-764-6317

Wayne State University
  School of Medicine
Dr. Silas Norman, Jr.
Assistant Dean for Admissions
540 E. Canfield Street 1310
Detroit, MI 48201
313-577-1466

MINNESOTA

Mayo Clinic College of Medicine
  Mayo Medical School
Dr. Patricia Barrier
Associate Dean for Student Affairs
200 First Street, SW
Rochester, MN 55905
507-284-3671

University of Minnesota
  Medical School
Dr. Lillian Repesh
Assoc. Dean for Admissions and
  Student Affairs, Duluth

Dr. Marilyn Becker
Director of Admissions, Twin Cities
MMC – 293
420 Delaware Street, SE
Minneapolis, MN 55455-0310
612-625-7977

MISSISSIPPI

University of Mississippi
School of Medicine
Dr. Steven Case
Associate Dean, Admissions
2500 N. State Street
Jackson, MS 39216-4505
601-984-5010

MISSOURI

A.T. Still University of Health
Sciences/Kirksville College of
Osteopathic Medicine [§]
Lori A. Haxton
Assistant to Vice President for
Admissions and Alumni Services
800 West Jefferson Street
Kirksville, MO 63501
866-626-2878 or 660-626-2237

Kansas City University of Medicine
and Biosciences [§]
Phil Byrne
Vice President Admissions
1750 Independence Avenue
Kansas City, MO 64106-1453
816-283-2350

University of Missouri–
Columbia School of Medicine
Judy Nolke
Admissions, Recruiting, Records
Coordinator
MA215,
Medical Science Building
One Hospital Drive
Columbia, MO 65212
573-882-9219

University of Missouri–Kansas City*
School of Medicine
Dr. Betty Drees
Dean
2411 Holmes Street
Kansas City, MO 64108
816-235-1870

Saint Louis University
School of Medicine
Dr. James Willmore
Associate Dean of Admissions
1402 S. Grand Boulevard
St. Louis, MO 63104
314-977-9870

Washington University
School of Medicine
Dr. W. Edwin Dodson
Associate Vice Chancellor and
Associate Dean for Admissions
660 S. Euclid Avenue, #8107
St. Louis, MO 63110
314-362-6857

NEBRASKA

Creighton University
School of Medicine
Dr. Henry Nipper
Assistant Dean for Admissions
Office of Medical Admissions
2500 California Plaza
Omaha, NE 68178
402-280-2799

University of Nebraska
College of Medicine
Dr. Jeffrey W. Hill
Associate Dean
Office of Admissions and Students
986585 Nebraska Medical Center
Omaha, NE 68198-6585
402-559-6140

NEVADA

University of Nevada
  School of Medicine
Cheryl Hug-English
Associate Dean for Admissions and
  Student Affairs
Office of Admissions and
  Student Affairs
Mail Stop 357
Reno, NV 89557-0129
775-784-6063

NEW HAMPSHIRE

Dartmouth Medical School
Andrew G. Welch
Director of Admissions
3 Rope Ferry Road
Hanover, NH 03755-1404
603-650-1505

NEW JERSEY

University of Medicine and
  Dentistry of NJ
  New Jersey Medical School
Dr. George F. Heinrich
Associate Dean for Admissions and
  Special Programs
185 S. Orange Avenue, C-653
Newark, NJ 07103
973-972-4631

University of Medicine and
  Dentistry of NJ
  Robert Wood Johnson Medical
  School
Dr. Carol A. Terregino
Associate Dean for Admissions
675 Hoes Lane
Piscataway, NJ 08854-5635
732-235-4576

University of Medicine and
  Dentistry of New Jersey
  School of Osteopathic Medicine [§]
Dr. Paul Kruger
Associate Dean for Academic
  Affairs
Office of Student Affairs, Suite 210
2nd Floor Academic Center
One Medical Center Drive
Stratford, NJ 08084
856-566-7050

NEW MEXICO

University of New Mexico
  School of Medicine
Dr. David G. Bear
Assistant Dean for Admissions
Office of Admissions
MSCO8 4690
Albuquerque, NM 87131-0001
505-272-4766

NEW YORK

Albany Medical College
Joanne H. Nanos
Director, Admissions and Student
  Records
Office of Admissions, MC3
47 New Scotland Avenue
Albany, NY 12208
518-262-5521

Albert Einstein College of Medicine
  of Yeshiva University
Noreen Kerrigan
Assistant Dean for Student
  Admissions
Jack & Pearl Resnick Campus
1300 Morris Park Avenue
Bronx, NY 10461
718-430-2106

Columbia University
  College of Physicians and
  Surgeons
Dr. Andrew G. Frantz
Associate Dean for Admissions
Admissions Office, Room 1-416
630 West 168th Street
New York, NY 10032
212-305-3595

Joan and Sanford I. Weill Medical
  College of Cornell University
Dr. Charles Bardes
Associate Dean and Chair,
  Admissions Committee
445 East 69th Street
New York, NY 10021
212-746-1067

Mt. Sinai School of Medicine of
  New York University
Dr. Scott Barnett
Assistant Dean for Admissions
Annenberg Building, Room 5-04
1 Gustave L. Levy Place
Box 1002
New York, NY 10029-6574
212-241-6696

New York College of Osteopathic
  Medicine of NY Institute of
  Technology §
Rodika Zaika
Director of Admissions
Northern Blvd.
Building 3, Room 203
Old Westbury, NY 11568
516-686-3700

New York Medical College
Dr. Fern Juster
Associate Dean and Chair,
  Admissions Committee
Admissions Building
Valhalla, NY 10595
914-594-4507

New York University
  School of Medicine
Joanne McGrath
Assistant Dean of Admissions
550 First Avenue
New York, NY 10016
212-263-5290

University of Rochester
  School of Medicine and Dentistry
Patricia Samuelson
Director of Admissions
601 Elmwood Avenue
Box 601-A
Rochester, NY 14642
585-275-4539

State University of New York –
  Downstate Medical Center
  College of Medicine
Dr. Eugene R. Fiegelson
Dean, Senior V.P. for Biomedical
  Education and Research
450 Clarkson Avenue, Box 60
Brooklyn, NY 11203-2098
718-270-2446

University at Buffalo
  School of Medicine and
  Biomedical Sciences
Dr. Charles Severin
Interim Senior Associate Dean of
  Medical Education
131 Biomed. Ed. Building
Buffalo, NY 14214-3013
716-829-3466

Stony Brook University
  School of Medicine
Health Sciences Center
Jack Fuhrer
Associate Dean for Admissions
Level 4
Stony Brook, NY 11794-8434
631-444-2113

State University of New York –
  Upstate Medical University
  College of Medicine
E. Gregory Keating, Ph.D.
Dean, Student Affairs
766 Irving Avenue
Syracuse, NY 13210
315-464-4570

NORTH CAROLINA

The Brody School of Medicine at
  East Carolina University
Dr. James G. Peden Jr.
Associate Dean for Admissions
Office of Admissions
Greenville, NC 27834
252-744-2202

Duke University
  School of Medicine
Dr. Brenda E. Armstrong
Associate Dean, Director of
  Admissions
P.O. Box 3710 DUMC
Durham, NC 27710
877-684-2985

University of North Carolina at
  Chapel Hill
  School of Medicine
Dr. Axalla Hoole
CB9500
Associate Dean, Admissions
121 MacNider Hall
Chapel Hill, NC 27599-9500
919-962-8331

Wake Forest University
  School of Medicine
Dr. Lewis H. Nelson, III
Associate Dean for Admissions
Medical Center Boulevard
Winston-Salem, NC 27157-1090
336-716-4264

NORTH DAKOTA

University of North Dakota*
  School of Medicine and Health
  Sciences
Judy L. DeMers
Associate Dean, Student Affairs &
  Admissions
501 N. Columbia Road, Box 9037
Grand Forks, ND 58202-9037
701-777-4221

OHIO

Case Western Reserve University
  School of Medicine
Dr. Amy Heneghan
Associate Dean for Admissions
10900 Euclid Avenue
Cleveland, OH 44106-4920
216-368-3450

University of Cincinnati
  College of Medicine
Dr. Laura Wexler
Associate Dean for Student Affairs
  and Admissions
P.O. Box 670552
Cincinnati, OH 45267-0552
513-558-7314

Medical University of Ohio
Dr. James F. Kleshinski
Associate Dean for Admissions
3045 Arlington Avenue
Toledo, OH 43614
419-383-4229

Northeastern Ohio Universities
  College of Medicine
Dr. Lois Margaret Nora
President and Dean
P.O. Box 95
Rootstown, OH 44272-0095
330-325-6270

Ohio State University
  College of Medicine and
  Public Health
Don Batisky, M.D.
Associate Dean of Admissions
155D Meiling Hall
370 W. Ninth Avenue
Columbus, OH 43210-1238
614-292-7137

Ohio University
  College of Osteopathic Medicine §
John Schriner, Ph.D.
Director of Admissions
102 Grosvenor Hall
Athens, OH 45701
740-593-4313

Wright State University
  School of Medicine
Dr. Paul G. Carlson
Associate Dean for Student Affairs/
  Admissions
P.O. Box 1751
Dayton, OH 45401-1751
937-775-2934

OKLAHOMA

Oklahoma State University
  College of Osteopathic Medicine §
Leah Haines
Assistant Director of Admissions
  and Recruitment
1111 W. 17th Street
Tulsa, OK 74107
918-582-1972

University of Oklahoma
  College of Medicine
Dotty Shaw Killam
Director for Admissions
P.O. Box 26901
Oklahoma City, OK 73190
405-271-2331

OREGON

Oregon Health & Science University
  School of Medicine
Dr. Cynthia Morris
Assistant Dean for Admissions
3181 SW Sam Jackson Park Road
Portland, OR 97239-3098
503-494-2998

PENNSYLVANIA

Lake Erie College of Osteopathic
  Medicine §
Elaine Morse
Admissions Coordinator
1858 W. Grandview Boulevard
Erie, PA 16509
814-866-6641

Jefferson Medical College
Dr. Clara Callahan
Dean of Students and Admissions
1015 Walnut Street, Suite 110
Philadelphia, PA 19107
215-955-6983

Drexel University
  College of Medicine
Dr. Cheryl A. Hanau
Assoc Dean for Admissions
2900 Queen Lane
Philadelphia, PA 19129
215-991-8202

Pennsylvania State University
  College of Medicine
Dr. Dwight Davis
Associate Dean for Student Affairs
  and Admissions
Suite H060
500 University Drive
P.O. Box 850
Hershey, PA 17033
717-531-8755

Philadelphia College of Osteopathic
  Medicine §
Carol Fox
Associate Vice President of
  Enrollment Management
4170 City Avenue
Philadelphia, PA 19131
215-871-6100

University of Pennsylvania
  School of Medicine
Gaye W. Sheffler
Director of Admissions and
  Financial Aid
Suite 100, Stemmler Hall
3450 Hamilton Walk
Philadelphia, PA 19104-6056
215-898-8001

University of Pittsburgh
  School of Medicine
Dr. Beth Piraino
Associate Dean of Admissions
518 Scaife Hall
Pittsburgh, PA 15261
412-648-9891

Temple University
  School of Medicine
Audrey B. Uknis, M.D.
Associate Dean for Admissions
Suite 305, Student Faculty Center
3340 N. Broad Street
Philadelphia, PA 19140
215-707-3656

PUERTO RICO

Universidad Central del Caribe
  School of Medicine
Dr. Jose Ginel Rodriguez
Dean of Medicine
Office of Admissions
P.O. Box 60-327
Bayamon, Puerto Rico 00960-6032
787-798-3001

Ponce School of Medicine
Dr. Carmen M. Mercado
Assistant Dean for Admissions
P.O. Box 7004
Ponce, Puerto Rico 00732-7004
787-840-2575

University of Puerto Rico
  School of Medicine
Margarita Rivera
Admissions Office
P.O. Box 365067
San Juan, Puerto Rico 00936-5067
787-758-2525

RHODE ISLAND

Brown University
  School of Medicine*
Dr. Philip Gruppuso
Associate Dean for Medical
  Education
Box G-A213
97 Waterman Street
Providence, RI 02912
401-863-2149

SOUTH CAROLINA

Medical University of South
  Carolina College of Medicine
Dr. Paul Underwood
Associate Dean, Admissions
96 Jonathan Lucas Street
Suite 601
P.O. Box 250617
Charleston, SC 29425
843-792-3283

University of South Carolina
  School of Medicine
Dr. Richard Hoppmann
Associate Dean for Medical
  Education and Academic Affairs
Columbia, SC 29208
803-733-3325

SOUTH DAKOTA

Sanford School of Medicine of the
  University of South Dakota
Dr. Paul Bunger
Dean Medical Student Affairs
414 E. Clark Street
Vermillion, SD 57069
605-677-6886

TENNESSEE

East Tennessee State University
  James H. Quillen College of
  Medicine
Edwin D. Taylor
Assistant Dean for Admissions and
  Records
P.O. Box 70580
Johnson City, TN 37614-1708
423-439-2033

Lincoln Memorial University—
DeBusk College of Osteopathic
  Medicine §
Paul Carney
Director of Admissions
6965 Cumberland Gap Parkway
Harrogate, TN 37752
423-869-7094

Meharry Medical College
  School of Medicine
Allen Mosley
Director/Admissions and Records
1005 Dr. D.B. Todd Boulevard
Nashville, TN 37208
615-327-6223

University of Tennessee
  Health Sciences Center
  College of Medicine
Dr. Hershel P. Wall
Dean (interim)
910 Madison Avenue
Memphis, TN 38163
901-448-5559

Vanderbilt University
  School of Medicine
Dr. Patricia Sagen
Director of Admissions
215 Light Hall
Nashville, TN 37232-0685
615-322-2145

TEXAS

Baylor College of Medicine
Dr. Lloyd Michael
Sr. Associate Dean of Admissions
Office of Admissions
One Baylor Plaza
Houston, TX 77030
713-798-4842

Texas A&M University System
  Health Sciences Center
  College of Medicine*
Filomeno G. Maldonado, Jr.
Assistant Dean of Admissions
159 Joe Reynolds Medical Bldg.
College Station, TX 77843-1114
979-845-7743

Texas College of Osteopathic
  Medicine §
Joel Daboub
Director, Admissions and Outreach
3500 Camp Bowie Blvd.
Fort Worth, TX 76107
817-735-2204

Texas Tech University*
  Health Sciences Center
  School of Medicine
Dr. Bernell Dalley
Associate Dean, Admissions and
  Minority Affairs
3601 4th Street
Lubbock, TX 79430
806-743-2297

University of Texas
  Southwestern Medical School
  at Dallas
Dr. Scott Wright
Director of Admissions
5323 Harry Hines Boulevard
Dallas, TX 75390-9162
214-648-5617

University of Texas*
  Medical School at Galveston
Dr. Lauree Thomas
Associate Dean, Admissions and
  Student Affairs
301 University Blvd.
Galveston, TX 77555-1317
409-772-1442

University of Texas*
  Medical School at Houston
Dr. Albert E. Gunn
Associate Dean for Admissions
6431 Fannin
MSB G.420
Houston, TX 77030
713-500-5116

University of Texas*
  Medical School at San Antonio
Dr. David J. Jones
Associate Dean, Admissions
7703 Floyd Curl Drive
San Antonio, TX 78229-3900
210-567-6080

UTAH

University of Utah
  School of Medicine
Dr. Wayne Samuelson
Associate Dean, Admissions
30 North 1900 East #1C029
Salt Lake City, UT 84132-2101
801-581-7498

VERMONT

University of Vermont
  College of Medicine
Tiffany Delaney
Director of Admissions
E-215 Given Building
89 Beaumont Avenue
Burlington, VT 05405
802-656-2154

VIRGINIA

Eastern Virginia Medical School
Susan L. Castora
Director of Admissions
700 West Onley Road
Norfolk, VA 23507
757-446-5812

Edward Via Virginia College of
  Osteopathic Medicine [§]
Megan Price
Director of Admissions
2265 Kraft Drive
Blacksburg, VA 24060
540-231-4000

Virginia Commonwealth University
  School of Medicine
Dr. Cynthia M. Heldberg
Assoc. Dean for Admissions
P.O. Box 980565
Richmond, VA 23298-0565
804-828-9629

University of Virginia
  School of Medicine
Dr. Beth A. Bailey
Assistant Dean for Admissions
Medical School Admissions Office
Box 800725
Charlotteville, VA 22908
434-924-5571

WASHINGTON

University of Washington
School of Medicine
Dr. Werner E. Sampson
Associate Dean for Admissions
Health Sciences Center A-300
Box 356340
Seattle, WA 98195-6340
206-543-7212

WEST VIRGINIA

Marshall University
Joan C. Edwards
School of Medicine
Cynthia A. Warren
Assistant Dean for Admissions and
Student Affairs
1600 Medical Center Drive
Huntington, WV 25701-3655
800-544-8514

West Virginia School of
Osteopathic Medicine [§]
Donna Varney
Director of Admissions
400 North Lee Street
Lewisburg, WV 24901
800-356-7836

West Virginia University
School of Medicine
Dr. David Morgan
Chair, Admissions Committee
P.O. Box 9111
Morgantown, WV 26506
304-293-2408

WISCONSIN

Medical College of Wisconsin
Michael Istwan
Director of Admissions
8701 Watertown Plank Road
Milwaukee, WI 53226
414-456-8246

University of Wisconsin
Medical School of Medicine and
Public Health
Lucy J. Wall
Assistant Dean for Admissions
Health Sciences Learning Center
750 Highland Avenue
Madison, WI 53705
608-263-4925

* Denotes non-AMCAS allopathic
medical school

[§] Denotes osteopathic medical
school

Personal Notes

Personal Notes

Personal Notes

Personal Notes

Personal Notes

Personal Notes